AGING WITH GRACE:

Redefining Beauty at Every Stage

BY

Rachel Ray

TABLE OF CONTENTS

INTRODUCTION

Aging with grace is a concept that encompasses embracing the process of growing older with dignity, confidence, and a positive mindset. It involves acknowledging and accepting the physical, emotional, and spiritual changes as we age while maintaining a sense of self-worth and inner beauty. Redefining beauty at every stage of life is crucial because societal standards often prioritize youthfulness and external appearance. However, true beauty goes beyond the surface and is rooted in wisdom, compassion, resilience, and self-acceptance. By redefining beauty, women can break free from the limitations imposed by societal norms and embrace their unique beauty at every age. Women can adopt several practices to embrace their beauty at every stage of life. Firstly, it is important to cultivate self-compassion and self-love. This involves treating oneself with kindness, embracing imperfections, and celebrating individuality. Women can enhance their overall sense of beauty and well-being by practicing self-care and nurturing their physical, emotional, and mental well-being. Another way to embrace beauty at every stage of life is to develop a positive body image. This entails shifting the focus from societal beauty ideals to honoring and appreciating one's body. By practicing gratitude for the body's strength, resilience, and the experiences it has facilitated throughout life, women can foster a sense of self-acceptance and love for their bodies. Additionally, women can embrace beauty by staying connected to their passions, interests, and personal growth. Engaging in activities that bring joy, learning new skills, and pursuing creative endeavors can create a sense of fulfillment and inner radiance. It is essential to prioritize self-expression and allow one's authentic self to shine through.

Furthermore, fostering meaningful connections and surrounding oneself with a supportive community can enhance women's sense of beauty and well-being. Building and nurturing relationships with loved ones, friends, and like-minded individuals can provide a sense of belonging and affirmation. Through these connections, women can find support, inspiration, and encouragement to embrace their beauty. Lastly, embracing beauty at every stage of life requires a shift in mindset. It involves challenging societal expectations and recognizing that beauty is not limited to a specific age or physical appearance. By cultivating a positive and empowered mindset, women can appreciate their worth, celebrate their accomplishments, and embrace the wisdom that comes with age. Embracing aging with grace and redefining beauty at every stage of life is an empowering act of self-love and liberation in a youth-obsessed world. By exploring the physical, emotional, mental, and spiritual aspects of aging, we uncover wisdom and beauty with each passing year. In the upcoming chapters, we navigate physical changes, emotions, cognitive function, and spiritual well-being to uncover the true meaning of beauty. Let's embark on a transformative journey to embrace our unique beauty and radiate an inner glow that illuminates every stage of life. The path to aging with grace awaits us, with insights into physical changes in the next chapter.

CHAPTER ONE

THE PHYSICAL CHANGES OF AGING

As women age, they embark on a transformative journey involving many physical changes. Grasping these changes and embracing them with grace and self-care is crucial for maintaining a sense of inner and outer beauty. One of the principal factors contributing to physical changes as women mature is the gradual decline in collagen production. Collagen, a protein that offers a framework for the skin's stability., gradually decreases. This decline leads to a reduction in skin thickness, elasticity, and resilience. The visible effects of collagen loss include fine lines, wrinkles, and sagging skin. It is important to note that collagen decline with aging is natural and influenced by various factors such as genetics, lifestyle, and environmental factors. Additionally, changes in skin elasticity play a significant role in the aging process. Elastin fibers, responsible for maintaining the skin's elasticity, become less abundant and resilient as we age. This can result in a loss of firmness and sagging, particularly in the face, neck, and arms. Understanding the intricacies of skin elasticity can help women develop targeted strategies to support and maintain the skin's firmness and youthful appearance. Hormonal shifts also contribute to physical changes experienced by women as they age. During menopause, for example, hormonal fluctuations occur, leading to a decline in estrogen levels. Estrogen is crucial in maintaining skin thickness, hydration, and overall health. As estrogen levels decrease, the skin may become drier, thinner, and more prone to irritation and sensitivity. These changes highlight the importance of adapting skincare routines and incorporating products that provide optimal hydration and nourishment.

To effectively manage and embrace these physical changes, developing practical strategies that nurture inner and outer beauty is crucial. Firstly, adopting a holistic approach to skincare is essential. This includes establishing a consistent skincare routine incorporating gentle cleansing, regular exfoliation, and moisturization to promote skin health and vitality. Daily application of sunscreen is crucial to shield the skin from sun damage, which can hasten aging and lead to skin problems such as wrinkles and age spots. Furthermore, maintaining a healthy lifestyle is key to supporting overall physical well-being and promoting the radiance that comes with age. A balanced diet with antioxidants, vitamins, and minerals nourishes the skin. Fruits, vegetables, whole grains, lean proteins, and healthy fats provide the essential nutrients for skin health. Regular physical activity is also crucial for managing and embracing physical changes. Exercise improves blood circulation, which helps deliver oxygen and nutrients to the skin, promoting a healthy complexion. Moreover, regular exercise enhances mood, reduces stress, and boosts overall well-being, further contributing to a sense of inner and outer beauty. In addition to external care, nurturing inner beauty is integral to embracing physical changes.

As women mature, they gain invaluable life experiences, wisdom, and a deeper understanding of themselves. This increased self-awareness and self-confidence radiate a unique beauty that transcends physical appearances. Cultivating self-love, practicing self-care, and embracing personal growth are transformative practices that enhance overall well-being and beauty. It is important to note that external attributes do not solely define beauty. True beauty encompasses kindness, compassion, resilience, and authenticity. Aging allows women to develop a deeper appreciation for these qualities, recognizing their immense value and power in shaping their lives and relationships.

CHAPTER TWO
THE EMOTIONAL CHANGES OF AGING

Aging is an innate and inescapable process that brings forth diverse alterations, not only in our physical appearance but also in our emotional well-being. As women age, they frequently encounter various emotional changes that can significantly impact their overall quality of life. Many factors, including hormonal fluctuations, life transitions, societal expectations, and personal experiences, can influence emotional changes during aging. It is imperative to acknowledge that each woman's journey is unique, and while some may navigate these changes with ease, others may face greater challenges. By comprehending the emotional landscape of aging, we can begin offering support and guidance to women who may be struggling. Psychology experts emphasize that women may experience a change in their emotional patterns as they grow older. This can manifest as increased introspection, heightened sensitivity, or greater emotional stability. While these changes can be unsettling, they also allow for personal growth and self-reflection. Throughout history, countless women have embraced the aging process gracefully and discovered newfound beauty in their later years. One such example is Sarah, a vibrant woman in her seventies who exudes confidence and joy. Like many others, Sarah experienced emotional changes as she aged, but she chose to perceive them as opportunities for self-discovery.

Sarah found solace in connecting with other women facing similar emotional challenges. Together, they formed a support group where they could candidly share their experiences, fears, and triumphs. Through these conversations, Sarah learned she was not alone in her journey and gained valuable insights into coping strategies and finding fulfillment.

Psychologists specializing in aging and emotionality underscore the importance of self-compassion during this transformative period. Dr. Emily Collins, a distinguished expert in the field, suggests that women should approach their emotional changes with curiosity and acceptance rather than judgment. By fostering self-compassion, women can navigate the ups and downs of aging with grace and resilience. Dr. Collins also emphasizes the significance of maintaining a robust support network. Engaging in meaningful relationships with friends, family, and community can provide emotional stability and a sense of belonging. Additionally, seeking professional support from therapists or counselors specializing in geriatric care can offer valuable guidance and tools to cope with emotional changes. Women can also draw inspiration from role models who have embraced aging gracefully. Icons like Helen Mirren, Jane Fonda, and Maya Angelou have publicly spoken about their experiences and the beauty they discovered in their later years. Their stories serve as reminders that age limitations don't prevent a satisfying life but rather provide an opportunity to redefine beauty and purpose. The emotional changes that occur as women age can be both arduous and gratifying. By comprehending these changes, embracing self-compassion, seeking support, and drawing inspiration from real stories of graceful aging, women can navigate this transformative period with grace and find happiness and fulfillment in every stage of life.

20

CHAPTER THREE

THE MENTAL CHANGES OF AGING

As we age, our cognitive function undergoes transformations that can impact various aspects of our mental well-being. As women advance in age, they may experience a variety of mental changes.These changes are subjective., and while some may face cognitive challenges, others may maintain mental acuity well into their later years. Generally, cognitive function tends to decline slightly with age, affecting memory, processing speed, and attention. Memory changes are among the most noticeable mental changes in aging women. This can include occasional forgetfulness or difficulty recalling certain details. However, it is essential to distinguish normal age-related memory changes from more severe conditions like dementia or Alzheimer's disease. Regular mental checkups with healthcare professionals can help identify any concerning cognitive decline. There are several strategies women can employ to maintain cognitive function as they age. Engaging in mentally stimulating activities is crucial. Reading books, solving puzzles, learning new skills, or participating in intellectually challenging hobbies can help keep the mind sharp and active. Physical exercise plays a significant role in maintaining cognitive function as well.These changes are subjective.It promotes better blood flow and the growth of new neurons in the brain. Combining physical activity with mentally stimulating tasks, such as dancing or playing a musical instrument, can have even more substantial benefits. Author and neuroscientist Dr. Lisa Johnson highlights the significance of maintaining a balanced lifestyle to support cognitive health. She recommends engaging in a variety of activities that challenge different cognitive abilities, such as problem-solving, creativity, and memory tasks. Dr. Elizabeth Thompson, a distinguished expert in geriatric psychology, emphasizes the importance of maintaining a positive mindset and reframing aging as a period of growth and wisdom. She suggests embracing a growth mindset, where women believe in their ability to continue learning and adapting throughout their lives.

Furthermore, a nutritious diet that includes foods rich in antioxidants, omega-3 fatty acids, and vitamins can support brain health. Maintaining social connections and staying socially engaged also contribute to cognitive well-being. Meaningful interactions with friends, family, and the community can provide mental stimulation, emotional support, and a sense of purpose. Women can take proactive steps to stay sharp and engaged in their later years. Continuing to acquire new knowledge, pursuing personal interests, and setting goals help stimulate the brain and foster a sense of achievement. Volunteering or engaging in community activities can provide a sense of purpose and keep women mentally and emotionally engaged. Utilizing relaxation methods like mindfulness or meditation can help lower stress and enhance mental clarity. Managing stress levels is essential because chronic stress has been linked to cognitive deterioration.

Additionally, good sleep is crucial for maintaining cognitive health. Creating a sleep-friendly environment and establishing a regular sleep schedule can help the brain function at its best.

CHAPTER FOUR

THE SPIRITUAL CHANGES OF AGING

Aging brings forth profound spiritual changes for women, marking a transformative phase in their lives. As they embark on this spiritual journey in their later years, women often experience a deepening of their spiritual beliefs, a yearning for meaning and purpose, and a desire to connect with their inner wisdom and strength. It's a time to look within, reflect, and embrace the beauty that comes out. Each woman's journey is distinctive within the tapestry of spiritual changes, shaped by her life experiences, values, and personal beliefs.

The aging process becomes a catalyst for self-discovery, prompting a reevaluation of priorities and a search for deeper significance. Existential questions arise, inviting women to explore the nature of existence and their place within the universe. Discovering meaning and purpose takes on heightened importance in the later years. It is an opportunity for women to engage in activities that resonate with their core values and passions, breathing life into their days. Some people find fulfillment in volunteering and putting their time and effort into causes they care about.

Others may immerse themselves in creative endeavors, expressing their innermost thoughts and emotions through art, music, or writing. The act of creation becomes a form of spiritual connection, allowing women to share their unique gifts with the world. In addition to external expressions of purpose, nurturing deep and meaningful connections becomes a vital source of spiritual fulfillment. Women find solace in fostering relationships with loved ones, engaging in heartfelt conversations, and offering support to others. Creating spaces for emotional intimacy and understanding nourishes the soul and reinforces the interconnectedness of all beings. Amidst the spiritual changes of aging, women often seek solace in practices that cultivate inner peace and connection. Meditation, prayer, or moments of quiet contemplation become gateways to the divine within. Women can cultivate presence, mindfulness, and a strong sense of gratitude for the present moment with the aid of these practices.

They offer a respite from the busyness of daily life, allowing women to reconnect with their inner selves and the greater spiritual tapestry of existence.

Connecting with inner wisdom and strength is an empowering aspect of the spiritual journey in aging. Women draw upon the wellspring of knowledge, insights, and resilience that have been honed throughout their lives. Self-reflection becomes a powerful tool for accessing this inner wisdom. Through journaling, introspection, and embracing solitude, women gain clarity and a deeper understanding of themselves. They come to recognize the lessons embedded within their life stories, both the triumphs and the challenges. Sharing these stories with others becomes a way of inspiring and empowering fellow travelers on the path. Renowned spiritual teachers and authors offer insights that can guide women on their spiritual journey.

CHAPTER FIVE
THE BEAUTY OF AGING

Beauty, often misunderstood and limited to external appearance, holds a deeper meaning that transcends age and societal expectations. It is a reflection of each woman's inner radiance, wisdom, and strength. Embracing beauty at every stage of life is a transformative journey that empowers women to redefine societal standards and inspire others to embrace their unique beauty. The true meaning of beauty lies in authenticity, self-acceptance, and the expression of one's inner light. It is a celebration of the multidimensional aspects that make each woman extraordinary. Beauty is not confined to youthful features or flawless skin; it embodies life experiences, resilience, and the lessons learned. Embracing beauty at every stage of life requires a shift in perspective and a redefinition of societal norms. It starts with recognizing that beauty is not bound by age but evolves and deepens with time. Women can rewrite the narrative and embrace the natural changes accompanying aging, finding beauty in the wrinkles, gray hair, and the stories on their faces. According to renowned author and activist Maya Angelou, a woman's beauty is not found in the clothes she wears, the shape she carries, or the way she combs her hair. The soul of a woman reflects her true beauty. This inspiring quote is a powerful reminder that true beauty comes from within and manifests in our demeanor, kindness, and love for others. Embracing one's beauty at every stage of life requires cultivating self-love and self-care. It involves nourishing the body, mind, and spirit. Physical well-being enhances confidence and vitality through exercise, nutritious food, and skincare routines. Mental and emotional well-being fostered through self-reflection, mindfulness practices, and nurturing relationships creates a strong foundation for embracing inner beauty.

Women who value their beauty set an excellent example for others. They defy social norms through self-acceptance and authenticity and inspire girls and women of all ages to appreciate their beauty. They spread inspiration and help others discover their inner beauty by sharing their knowledge, experiences, and stories. Embracing the beauty of aging is also about reframing societal beauty standards and advocating for inclusivity. It is about celebrating diversity and the richness that comes from women of different backgrounds, cultures, and experiences. Through this collective celebration, we create a world where every woman feels seen, valued, and beautiful in her own right.

As women age, they can redefine beauty on their terms. They can explore new styles, experiment with fashion and makeup, and express their individuality in ways that make them feel confident and empowered. It is a time to embrace personal preferences and let go of societal expectations.

Moreover, the beauty of aging lies in the wisdom and experience women have gained over the years. It is through the challenges faced, and the lessons learned that a woman's character deepens and her beauty shines. Every wrinkle tells a story of resilience, every gray hair a badge of wisdom earned. These physical changes become symbols of strength and endurance, reflecting a life well-lived. Women can encourage others to value their beauty by sharing their experiences and stories. By speaking openly about their journey of self-acceptance and self-love, they can help others recognize the inherent beauty within themselves. Kindness, compassion, and selflessness further enhance the beauty that radiates from within.

Celebrating and uplifting women of all ages is essential, recognizing that beauty knows no boundaries. Through intergenerational connections, women can inspire and learn from one another. Younger generations can look to older women as role models, appreciating their wisdom and grace. That comes with age. In turn, older women can find inspiration and rejuvenation through the energy and enthusiasm of the younger generations. The true meaning of beauty transcends age and external appearance. It resides within the depth of each woman's soul, reflecting her authenticity, wisdom, and resilience. Embracing beauty at every stage of life involves a shift in perspective, self-love, and self-care. By embracing their beauty, women inspire others to do the same, challenging societal norms and celebrating the richness of diversity. Let us all embrace the beauty of aging and shine our inner light for the world to see.

CONCLUSION

Finally, the journey of Women are urged to accept and appreciate their beauty throughout their entire life, as "aging with grace" is emphasized as an important goal. Throughout the chapters of this book, we have explored the physical, emotional, mental, and spiritual changes that occur as women age. We have discussed strategies for managing these changes, finding happiness and fulfillment, and maintaining cognitive function. Now, let us delve into the essence of beauty and how women can truly embrace it as they navigate their later years. At its core, beauty extends far beyond societal standards and external appearance. It is a reflection of inner radiance, strength, and authenticity. Embracing beauty at every stage of life requires a shift in perspective, a celebration of each woman's unique journey. It is a call to cherish and honor one's wisdom and experiences as valuable assets that contribute to one's beauty. True beauty lies in embracing oneself fully, with all the physical, emotional, and spiritual changes that accompany aging. It is about self-acceptance and self-love, nurturing a deep connection with one's inner essence. By embracing the physical changes, women can view them as symbols of resilience and the stories that have shaped their lives. Moreover, beauty is not an isolated experience but a gift to be shared with others. Women have the power to inspire those around them, encouraging them to embrace their unique beauty. By being authentic and unapologetic in their self-expression, women can create a ripple effect, transforming societal perceptions of beauty and promoting inclusivity and self-acceptance. Women must prioritize self-care and well-being to embrace beauty at every stage of life. This includes nourishing the mind, body, and spirit through mindfulness, self-reflection, and self-compassion. Engaging in activities that bring joy, pursuing passions, and fostering meaningful connections are all vital aspects of this journey. As we conclude this exploration of aging with grace and redefining beauty, I invite every woman to embark on her journey of self-discovery and self-acceptance. Embrace the physical, emotional, mental, and spiritual changes that come with age, recognizing them as opportunities for growth and transformation Remember, beauty knows no boundaries of age or societal expectations. It is a radiant force that emanates from within and shines brightly throughout the different chapters of life. Embrace your beauty, embrace your journey, and let us create a world that honors and celebrates the beauty of aging.

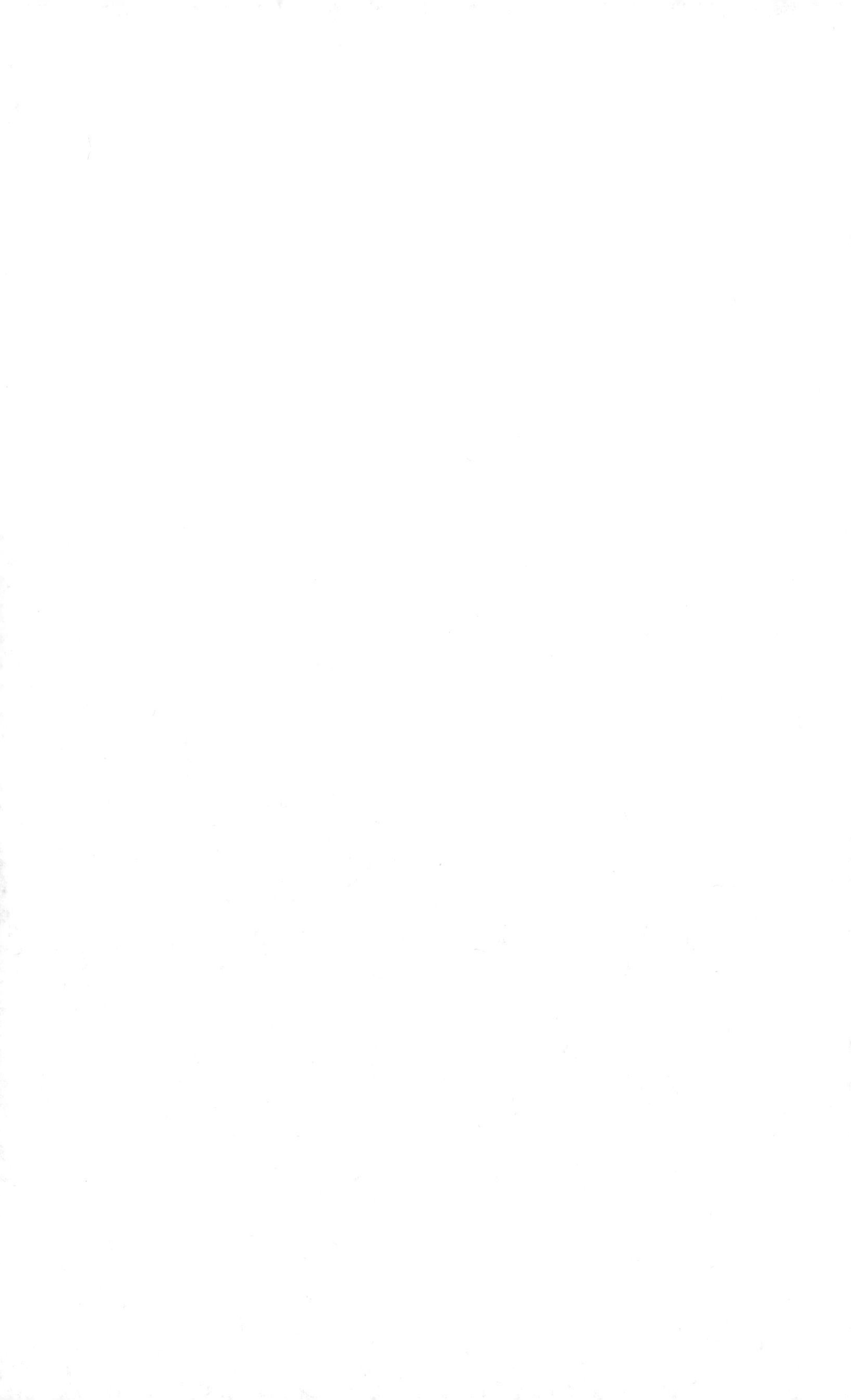

9 798397 634335